Stretching
Without
Pain

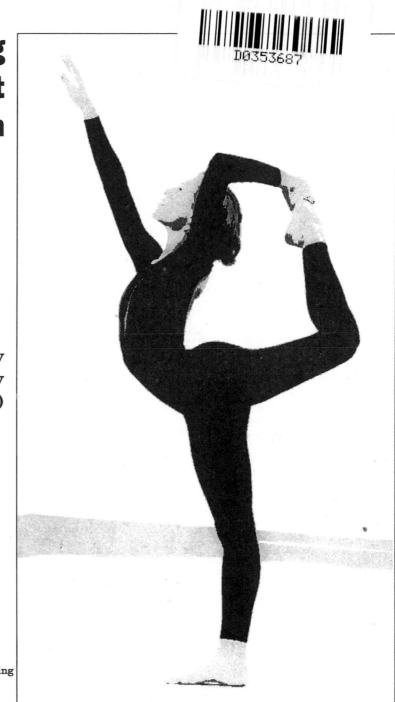

by
W Paul Blakey
LCSP(DO)

Twin Eagles Educational & Healing
Institute in association with
Bibliotek Books.

Dedication

Stretching Without Pain has had an elephantine gestation. After writing and illustrating The Muscle Book I decided to move back to Canada, to western BC, where I am presently living. This move, with my family, took more effort than I could ever have imagined. So despite the success of The Muscle Book and requests for a second book from my publisher and readers, I was unable to embark seriously on this task until 1994, two and a half years after leaving England.

I would like to thank my wife, Nicola who has supported me emotionally and financially during the time it has taken me to complete this project. And Gemma for proof reading. Also I would like to thank Phylis Austin and all the folks who sent me information via Internet. And Alison Denham the young dancer/model pictured in the following pages.

Published by:
Twin Eagles Educational & Healing Institute in association with **Bibliotek Books.**
19 Warwick Rd
Stafford
ST17 4PD

Disclaimer

The author and publisher of this material are not liable or responsible to any person for any damage caused or alleged to be caused directly or indirectly by the information contained in this book.

If you are in any doubt, consult a physician.

Contents

Stretching Without Pain

Reading without pain.

Proprioception: pertaining to, or made active by, stimuli arising from movement in the tissues.

In this book I am attempting to explain the neuro-physiology of stretching. To reveal the elegant system of checks and balances that we call proprioception.

I have designed this book to be read sequentially, so that each packet of information leads to the next, much as a house is built upon a firm foundation.

So we begin by looking at the types of joints there are in the body, particularly the synovial joints. This leads on to an examination of our normal range of motion. It is important to realize that your normal joint mobility is more than enough for your needs.

A look at connective tissue, including ligaments, tendons and fascia will tell you what stretches and what does not stretch. And once you understand this you are ready to learn how your muscles are 'set' by certain protective nerve cells.

An introduction to mental/emotional considerations comes next. Followed by information about warming up and how you can stretch more efficiently by knowing when to stretch and in what order.

Then descriptions of the different types of stretching, including pages detailing suggested stretching techniques.

Then you are ready for a tour through the Flexibility Supermarket.

And finally we talk about War Zones. Areas of the body that act like armour or walled cities.

If you read carefully and take your time to think about what is being said, you should be able to understand the principles behind safe, painless, yet amazingly efficient stretching. If you are utilizing these techniques to improve your own flexibility, or if you are a teacher, then please remember this rule of thumb...

If it hurts, you are doing something wrong.

4

Anatomical Terminology.

Abduction: means taking or drawing away.
Adduction: means drawing inward.
Extension: means stretching out.
Flexion: means bending or folding.
Rotation: means turning round, like a wheel.

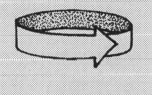

Anterior: means in front.
Frontal: this plane divides the body into front/back.
Inferior: means lower, closer to the feet.
Lateral: means to the side, going away from the midline.
Median: is the midline plane dividing the body into left/right.
Posterior: means behind.
Superior: means above, closer to the head.
Transverse: this plane divides the body into upper/lower.

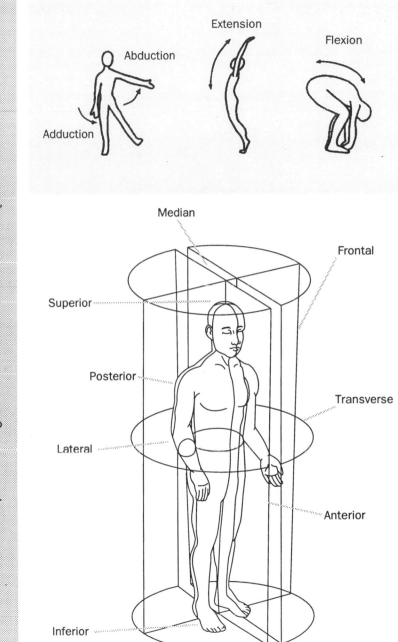

Stretching Without Pain

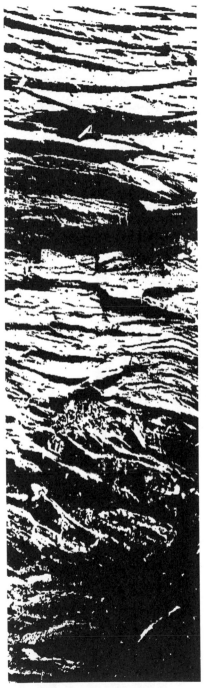

Description of Joints

Structure of a Synovial Joint

Normal Range of Motion

Neck
Shoulder
Elbow
Wrist
Spine
Hip
Knee
Ankle

Types of Flexibility

Strength and Flexibility

Warning

Description of joints

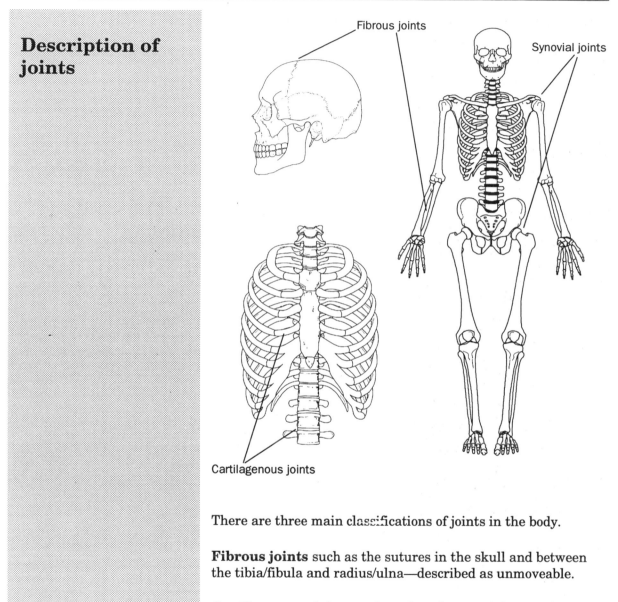

Fibrous joints

Synovial joints

Cartilagenous joints

There are three main classifications of joints in the body.

Fibrous joints such as the sutures in the skull and between the tibia/fibula and radius/ulna—described as unmoveable.

Cartilagenous joints such as those between the vertebrae or between the ribs/sternum—described as slightly moveable.

Synovial joints which are freely moveable joints and the ones we will be examining in regard to flexibility.

Structure of a synovial joint

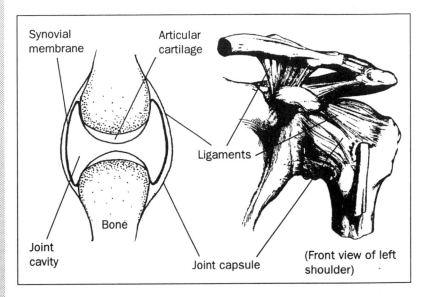

Synovial membrane

Articular cartilage

Ligaments

Bone

Joint cavity

Joint capsule

(Front view of left shoulder)

Joint capsule—this is a sleeve-like extension of the periosteum (bone covering) of each of the articulating bones. A capsule is formed which creates a complete casing around the ends of both bones, joining them together.

Synovial membrane—this is a slippery membrane that lines the inner surface of the joint capsule. It attaches to the margins of the articular cartilage and secretes synovial fluid which acts as a lubricant and nourishes the interior of the joint.

Articular cartilage—this covers and cushions the two end surfaces of each bone.

Joint cavity—this is the space between the two bones. It is this free space that allows freedom of movement.

Menisci—articular cartilage between some joints, the most commonly injured ones being the knee cartilages.

Ligaments—strong cords of dense white fibrous tissue that bind the two joints firmly together.

Normal Range of Motion

If you test one joint against another you should quickly see that 1; your joint mobility is by no means symmetrical and 2; that your normal range of motion is more than enough for your needs.

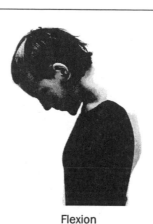

Flexion

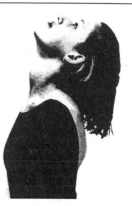

Extension

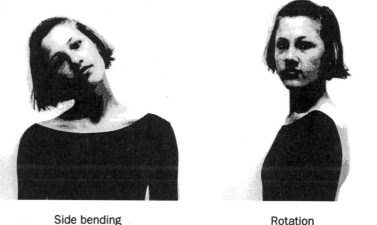

Side bending

Rotation

Neck

You should be able to:
>   touch your chest with your chin (flexion 70-90°)
>   point your chin to the sky (extension 55°)
>   bring your ear close to your shoulder (side bending 35°)
>   turn head left and right (rotation 70° each side)

Normal Range of Motion

There is no need to stretch ligaments to increase your mobility. The trick is in training your muscles to allow the joints to reach their *normal* mobility.

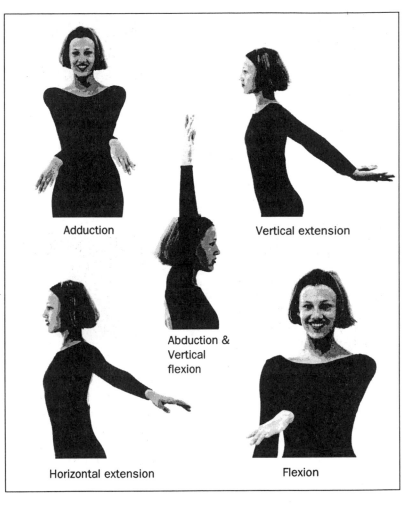

Adduction

Vertical extension

Abduction & Vertical flexion

Horizontal extension

Flexion

Shoulder

You should be able to:
  raise your arm straight up (abduction 180°)
  bring arm towards midline of your body (adduction 45°)
  lift arm horizontally backwards (extension 45°)
  lift arm horizontally forwards (flexion 130°)
  raise arm straight backwards (vertical extension 60°)
  raise arm straight forwards (vertical flexion 180°)

Normal Range of Motion

Flexible, according to the dictionary means *easily bent*. If you remember this when you are stretching you should start to understand that increasing flexibility does not mean increasing the strain on your joints, it means making them easy to bend.

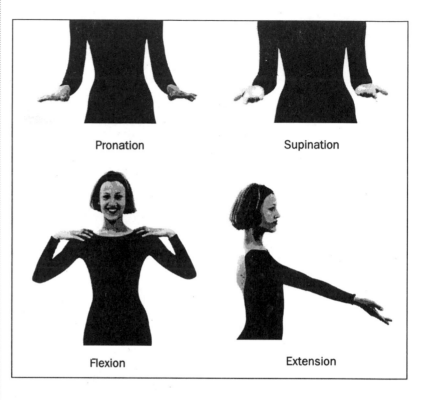

Pronation

Supination

Flexion

Extension

There is a common difference between men and women's elbows due to the shape of the humerus, which in straighten beyond 180°. more common in women fact.

the hollow in the posterior of women allows the arm to Overstretching the elbow is because of this anatomical

Hollow

Elbow

You should be able to:

       straighten your lower arm (extension 180°)
       bring your lower arm to your biceps (flexion 150°)
       turn your hand palm upwards (supination 90°)
       turn your hand palm downwards (pronation 90°)

Normal Range of Motion

What affects flexibility?

Internal Influences:

- the type of joint
- resistance within the joint
- elasticity of muscle tissue (is there any scar tissue?)
- elasticity of ligaments and tendons (not much)
- elasticity of skin
- ability to relax muscles
- temperature of joint and surrounding tissues (higher body temperatures aid flexibility)
- mental attitude

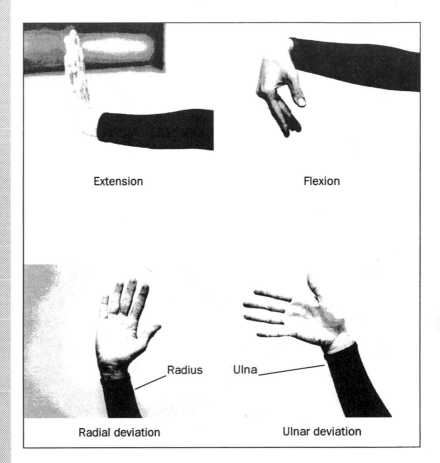

Extension   Flexion

Radius   Ulna

Radial deviation   Ulnar deviation

Wrist

You should be able to:
>   bend wrist as if gripping (flexion 80-90°)
>   bend wrist as if pushing (extension 70°)
>   bend wrist so thumb nears radius (radial deviation 20°)
>   bend wrist so fingers near ulna (ulnar deviation 30-50°)

Normal Range of Motion

External Influences:

- outside temperature
- time of day
- stage of recovery from injury
- age
- gender
- ability
- commitment
- mental attitude of those around you
- clothing or equipment

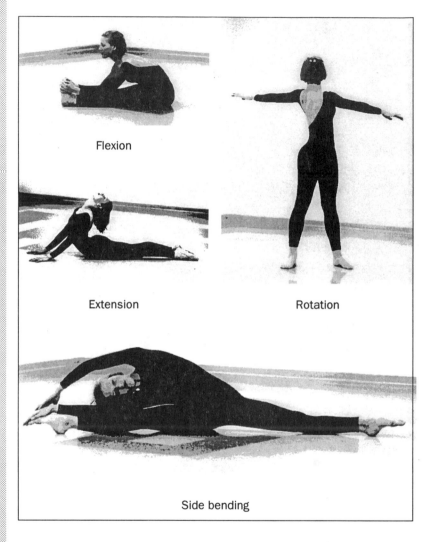

Flexion

Extension

Rotation

Side bending

Spine

You should be able to:
> bend forward at the waist (flexion 75°)
> bend backward at the waist (extension 30°)
> bend to the side (side bending 35°)
> rotate left and right (rotation 45°)

Normal Range of Motion

What affects flexibility the most?

(In order of most resistance to least).

- **Joint capsule and ligaments—47%**
- **Muscle fascia—41%**
- **Tendons—10%**
- **Skin—2%**

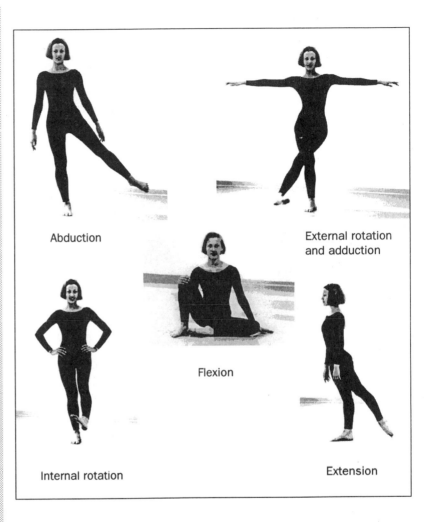

Abduction

External rotation and adduction

Flexion

Internal rotation

Extension

Hip

You should be able to:

 flex knee and bring thigh to abdomen (flexion 110-130°)
 move thigh backwards with pelvis still (extension 30°)
 move thigh away from midline (abduction 45-50°)
 move thigh toward and across midline (adduction 20-30°)
 rotate leg outwards (external rotation 45°)
 rotate leg inwards (internal rotation 40°)

Normal Range of Motion

Though it seems the joint capsule and ligaments exert the most influence on flexibility it is the muscle fascia which is best to work on. This is because the muscle fascia contains much more elastic tissue, whereas ligaments and tendons have almost no elastic tissue and if you do succeed in painfully causing them to stretch, they will not have the ability to regain their normal length and thus lead to future injury due to excess mobility.

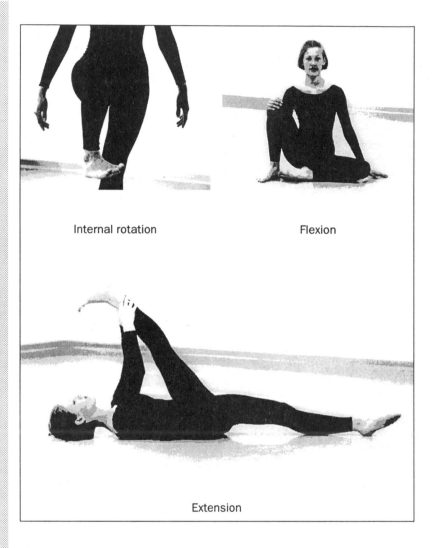

Internal rotation · Flexion

Extension

Knee

You should be able to:
>   touch calf muscle to hamstring (flexion 130°)
>   straighten knee (extension 15°)
>   rotate lower leg inwards (internal rotation 10°)

Normal Range of Motion

Age is also an important factor, not so much because of general tissue changes that come with age, but because of the injuries and scar tissue and faulty neuromuscular programming that accompanies age.

And *fixed mental attitudes.*

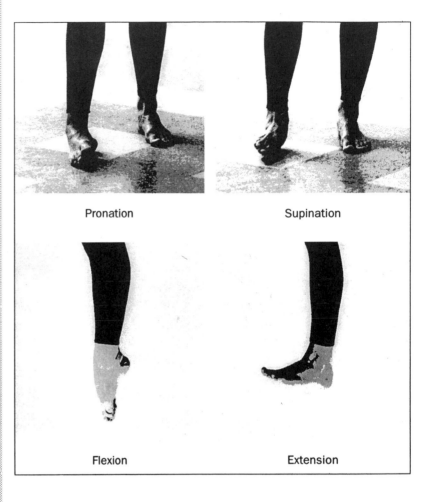

Pronation   Supination

Flexion   Extension

Ankle

You should be able to:
bend ankle so toes point up (dorsiflexion 20°)
bend ankle so toes point down (flexion 45°)
turn foot sole upwards (inversion 30°)
turn foot sole outwards (eversion 20°)

Stretching Without Pain

Types of Flexibility

The hardest of these to develop is static-active flexibility.

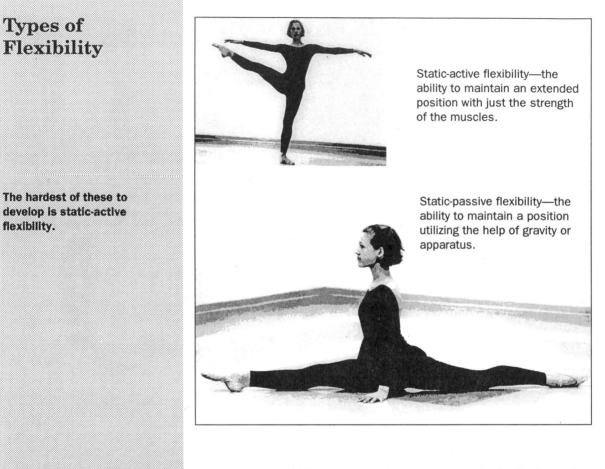

Static-active flexibility—the ability to maintain an extended position with just the strength of the muscles.

Static-passive flexibility—the ability to maintain a position utilizing the help of gravity or apparatus.

Dynamic flexibility—is the ability to bring the limb through a complete range of movement. (An example of this would be high kicks to the front, side or back).

Static-active flexibility—the ability to maintain an extended position with just the strength of the muscles. (An example would be holding the leg in front, side or behind).

Static-passive flexibility—the ability to maintain a position utilizing the help of gravity or apparatus. (An example would be doing the splits, or holding your leg up with your arm or by placing it on a supporting surface).

Strength and Flexibility

A muscle that can lengthen before it contracts can contract with more force. This is obvious if you look at any throwing sport such as baseball or javelin. The more stretch there is in the pectoral muscles, the longer and faster the throw. Similarly with runners, the longer the stride, the faster they go.

For activities that demand both strength and suppleness the key is to train for both.

If the training workout involves dynamic stretches, such as dance, then there is less need to worry about muscle shortening. Though I would suggest as a rule of thumb that every strength move should be followed by an opposing stretch.

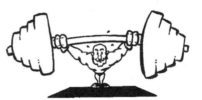

But especially if you do any weight training, it is important to stretch. This is because most weight training overloads and fatigues the muscles, leaving them pumped full of fluids, including large quantities of lactic acid and other muscle metabolism by-products. If the muscle is not stretched afterwards it tends to retain a decreased range of motion (almost as if it 'forgets' how to lengthen). So stretching helps to remove harmful by-products and prevents shortening.

Heavy workouts tend to damage muscle tissue. Static stretching is advised in order to prevent the tissues healing at a shorter length.

Naturally flexible people should do just the opposite. They should stretch first and do strength exercises second. If the connective tissue is weak then it is necessary to strengthen the muscles. The best type of work is dynamic strength training. Lots of repetitions through the full range of movement. Again dance training is a superb example.

Stretching Without Pain

Once your muscles have reached their maximum length, continuing stretching only stretches the ligaments and stresses the tendons. Ligaments will tear when stretched beyond a 6% increase over normal length and tendons are not supposed to stretch at all. Excess stretching will only result in destabilized joints which are much more likely to be injured.

Young gymnasts are probably the most vulnerable in this regard. Especially the lower lumbar joints, which can be permanently damaged by excessive back bending. Be careful—be thoughtful! Look at how a young person recovers from a back bend. If the movement is not smooth and graceful then there is probably some pain involved, and if there is pain then there is probably over stretching, and if there is over stretching there is an accident just waiting to happen.

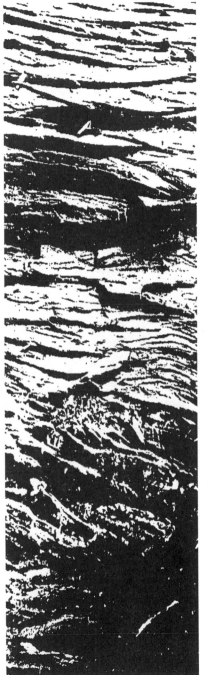

Connective Tissue

Ligaments

White fibrous tissue
Yellow elastic tissue

Tendons

Joint Capsule

Fascia

Superficial fascia
Deep fascia
Fascial sheaths

Stretching Without Pain

Connective Tissue

Elastic: having a tendency to recover the original form or size.

Collagen: a protein in fibrous connective tissue, readily turned into gelatine - from Gk. *to become glue.*

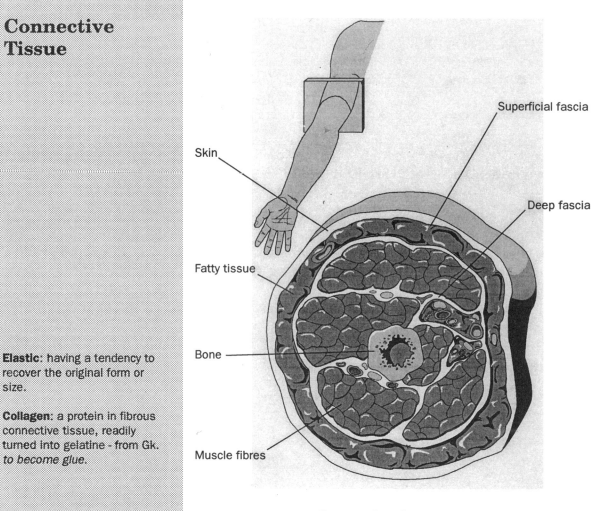

Cross section of upper arm.

Muscle fibre is surrounded by connective tissue. This tissue is comprised of a base substance and two types of fibre, collagenous and elastic. The collagenous fibre provides strength and the elastic fibre provides elasticity. The base substance (mucopolysaccharide) acts as both a lubricant and a glue.

Ligaments

If a ligament is over stretched it will usually return to its original length after a few weeks rest.

However, if the same ligament is repeatedly over stretched it will become slack and non-functional. The joint is then loosened and injury is more likely to happen.

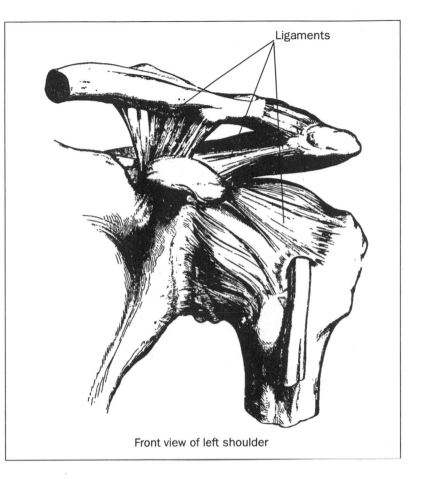

Ligaments

Front view of left shoulder

Ligaments are composed mainly of bundles of *white fibrous tissue* placed parallel with or closely interlaced with one another which creates a white, shining, silvery effect. A ligament is pliant and flexible so as to allow good freedom of movement, but is also strong, tough and inextensible (does not stretch). This type of ligament supports most joints.

Some ligaments are composed of *yellow elastic tissue* and in these cases the elasticity is intended to act as a substitute for muscular power. (Example: ligamenta subflava connecting adjacent arches of the vertebrae).

23

Stretching Without Pain

White Fibrous and Yellow Elastic tissue

Most ligaments are not designed to stretch. If they are stretched more than 6% past their normal length, they will tear. So there is no sense in trying to stretch them to increase flexibility. Your normal range of motion is more than adequate. (See normal range of motion.)

The white fibres are arranged in waving bands or bundles. They have a tendency to split up longitudinally but the individual fibres are unbranched and never join other fibres.

The yellow elastic fibres form bold wide curves and freely join with each other. They tend to curl up at the end.

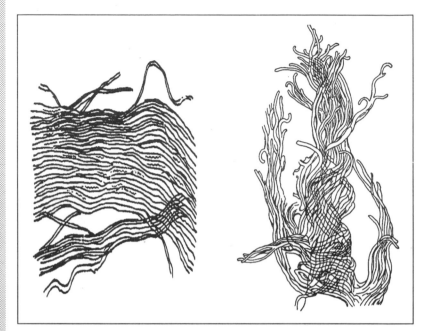

White fibrous tissue

The white fibres predominate in this tissue. To the naked eye it has the appearance of silvery-white glistening fibres covered over with a quantity of loose tissue that binds the fibres together and carries the blood vessels. It is not elastic and only stretches slightly. However, it is very strong and usually the bone it is attached to will fracture before the fibrous tissue gives way. In ligaments and tendons the bundles of tissue run parallel with each other.

Yellow elastic tissue

This tissue is very elastic and can be stretched considerably. And because it is elastic, it will return to its original length after stretching, just like a rubber band. It is a connective tissue that contains almost exclusively yellow elastic fibres. Found in the ligamenta subflava, vocal chords, trachea, bronchi, blood vessels (particularly arteries) and thyro-hyoid, crico-hyoid and stylo-hyoid ligaments.

Tendons

The connective tissue surrounding the muscle extends into the white fibrous tissue that is the tendon. Thus elastic tissue and non-elastic tissue make a seamless join.

As you get older the collagen changes, becoming more rigid and liable to tear.

Tendons do NOT stretch!

White, glistening, fibrous cords, varying in length and thickness. Sometimes round, sometimes flattened, very strong and not at all elastic. Made of white fibrous tissue, the fibres are laid down in an undulating path parallel to each other. Sparingly supplied with blood vessels, the smaller tendons having none at all in the interior. Nerves are only present in the larger tendons such as the Achilles tendon.

Aponeuroses are flattened or ribbon-shaped tendons. Pearly white, iridescent, glistening. Mostly without nerves or only sparingly supplied with blood vessels.

Tendons and aponeuroses join muscles to bone. In most cases the actual join is so smooth as to be almost invisible. But where the muscle joins the tendon at an angle the joining is more noticeable.

Tendons are less flexible than ligaments, having no elasticity at all. If a tendon is extended only four percent beyond its normal length, it will be irreversibly deformed.

Aponeurosis

Achilles tendon

Fascia

Fascia: from Latin; meaning a band, or bandage.

This is a microscopic view of fibro-areolar tissue of variable thickness and strength found in all regions of the body. There are two main divisions, superficial and deep.

Areolar tissue

So called because it is full of open spaces (areolae). This makes it easy to inject air or fluid into this tissue. This tissue acts as a general binder for all other tissues but because it is so easily permeable it allows fluids to move through it fairly easily. It is one of the most extensively distributed of all tissues. Found beneath the skin in a continuous layer all over the body. It is found between muscles, vessels and nerves, forming investing sheaths for them and connecting them with surrounding structures. In addition it is found in the interior of organs, binding the hollow viscera and the fibres of muscles.

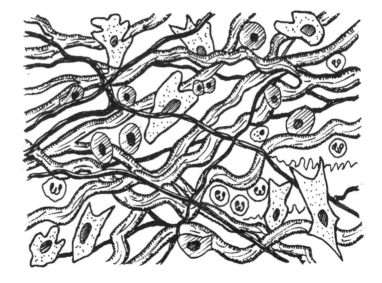

To the naked eye areolar tissue looks like spun silk. When stretched out it is seen to consist of delicate soft elastic threads interlaced with each other in every direction and forming a network of extreme delicacy. It is composed of white fibres and elastic fibres intercrossing in all directions and united by a cement or ground substance, the matrix. Within this matrix lie connective tissue corpuscles which contain the protoplasm out of which the whole is developed and regenerated.

Fascia Superficial and Deep

Fascial Sheaths

There are three categories of sheath, named according to where they are found in the muscles.

Epimysium: 'epi' means on or over, so this is the outermost sheath that binds all of the individual muscle fibres and the groups of these fibres together.

Perimysium: 'peri' means around, so this is the sheath that binds groups of individual muscle fibres.

Endomysium: 'endo' means inner or inside, so this is the sheath of each individual muscle fibre.

Superficial fascia.

Found immediately beneath the skin over almost the entire surface of the body. It connects the skin to adjacent parts, facilitates movement of the skin and serves as a soft medium for the passage of vessels and nerves to the skin. It also retains the warmth of the body due to the fat (adipose tissue) contained within its areolae.

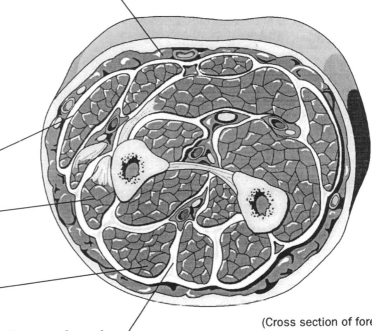

(Cross section of forearm)

Deep fascia.

A dense, inelastic fibrous membrane, forming sheaths for the muscles and giving them broad surfaces for attachment. Consists of shining tendinous fibres placed parallel with each other. The deep fasciae assist muscles in their action by the degree of tension and pressure they make upon their surface. In certain situations this is increased and regulated by muscular action such as the Tensor Fascia Lata, Gluteus Maximus in the thigh and the Biceps in the arm, also the Palmaris Longus of the hand.

Stretching Without Pain

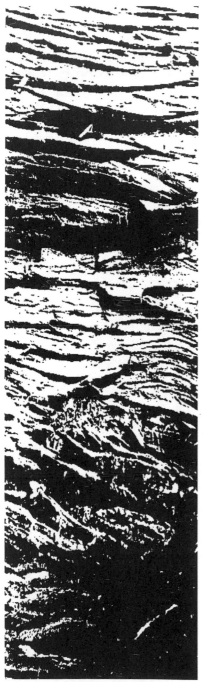

Muscle Tissue

How Muscles Contract

Neuromuscular (the nerve circuits)
Physiology (the structures involved)

Stretch Receptors

Inhibiting Contraction

Definition of Muscle Groups

Agonists/Prime Movers
Antagonists
Synergists
Fixators

Brain-Muscle Links

Muscle Tissue

There are three types of muscle, smooth, striped and cardiac.

From its normal resting length a muscle can be contracted to 70% or stretched to 130%.

In relation to stretching we will be concentrating on striped, or skeletal muscle. Cardiac muscle is heart muscle and smooth muscle is found mainly in the viscera, and neither need to be stretched.

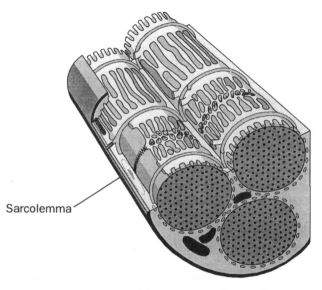

Sarcolemma

Muscle Fibre (magnified)

Striped or skeletal muscle when seen under a microscope has a striped appearance and is arranged in bundles mostly parallel to each other and converging towards the tendons.

A muscle fibre consists of a soft, contractile substance enclosed in a tubular sheath. This sheath is called the sarcolemma. Within this sheath are thousands of tiny threads that can contract and elongate. These are in turn made up of millions of bands called sarcomeres and each of these is made up of filaments called myofilaments. These myofilaments consist of contractile proteins. There are two kinds of protein, actin and myosin; the attraction these two proteins have for each other causes the muscle fibre to contract.

The tubular sheath is quite strong, and even when the muscle fibre within the sheath tears, the sheath will often stay intact.

How Muscles Contract

Neuromuscular (the nerve circuits).

Physiology (the process involved).

Medullated fibres are enclosed within a delicate membrane, which acts as a protective sheath/insulator.

Neuromuscular

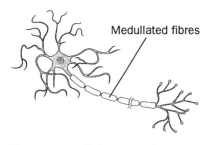

Medullated fibres

Nerves supplying muscle fibres are derived from the cerebro-spinal nerves and are composed of mainly medullated fibres. The nerve, after entering the sheath of the muscle, breaks up into fibres, or bundles of fibres, which form plexuses and gradually divide until a single nerve fibre enters a muscle fibre. Within the muscle fibre the nerve expands and creates what has been described as a motor-end-plate. The protective coating disappears as the nerve fibre becomes one with the muscle fibre.

The place where the nerve and muscle meet is called the neuromuscular junction. An electrical signal crossing this junction stimulates the flow of calcium which causes the myofilaments to slide across one another. When this happens the sarcomere shortens and force is generated. Billions of sarcomeres shortening causes a contraction of the entire muscle fibre.

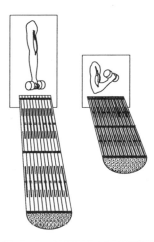

A muscle fibre contracts completely or not at all. The way we are able to vary the amount of contraction relative to the load is by recruiting more muscle fibres as the load increases. Think of it this way; you have a thousand men ready to pull on a rope and you number them from 1 to 1000. When the load they are pulling is not too great then only the first 250 are asked to pull, but they all have to pull with all their might. As the load increases, the next 250 are called in to help, and then another 250 and then another, until all 1000 are working. As you can see, numbers 750—1000 don't work very often, only when the load is near the limit.

Stretching Without Pain

Neuromuscular

Proprioceptive: pertaining to, made active by stimuli arising from movement in the tissues.

Muscle spindles are connected parallel to other muscle cells, in the belly of the muscle. They passively follow the movement of the cells they are attached to. If the muscle cell stretches then so does the spindle cell.

Tapping the patellar ligament below the kneecap causes the thigh muscle to stretch unexpectedly. The resulting contraction is due to the activity of the spindle cells. The period of time between the tap and the movement of the leg is the time it takes for the nerve impulse to travel from the spindle cells to the spinal cord and back to the muscle cells.

Crucial to the neural control of muscles is the feedback system which enables the central nervous system to accomodate different body needs. In relation to stretching, the most important nerves are the proprioceptors.

Proprioceptors are found in all nerve endings of the joints, muscles and tendons. The ones related to stretching are found in the tendons and in the muscle fibres.

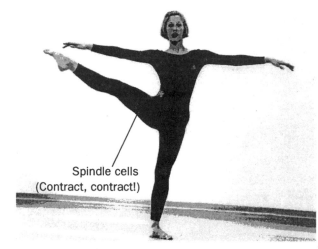

Spindle cells
(Contract, contract!)

Spindle cells, or stretch receptors, are found in the belly of the muscle. These tell when the muscle is lengthening and send messages telling the muscle to contract, if they go beyond a certain, pre-determined length, or if they try to lengthen too quickly. There are two types of stretch receptor; one measures magnitude and the other measures speed. Going too far, too fast will frighten a muscle into a protective contraction. This is why successful flexibility training starts slowly, building towards dynamic stretching, as the receptors are *re-educated*.

The stretch receptors also inhibit the opposing muscle, allowing the agonist/antagonist loop to further protect the muscle being stretched. (If for example the hamstring was being stretched by attempting a high front kick, the stretch receptors would stimulate the hamstrings to contract, while at the same time inhibiting the lifting muscle, the quadriceps. This would effectively stop the upward movement of the leg).

Stretch Receptors

It is most important to realize that stretch training is actually re-training the neuromuscular components, rather than artificially trying to distort connective tissue.

Golgi tendon receptors are located near the end of the muscle fibre, where fibre becomes tendon. When the muscle contracts, the tendon receptors measure the tension on the tendons and send messages telling the muscle to relax if the tension reaches beyond a certain pre-determined level.

This is necessary to prevent injury from excessive force being applied to the tendons, ligaments and muscles. This only happens when the golgi signals to the spinal cord are stronger than the signals from the spindle cells. (You can imagine the spindles all yelling 'contract, contract' and the golgi receptors yelling, 'relax, relax').

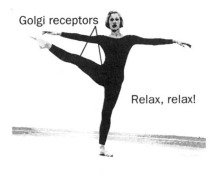

Golgi receptors

Relax, relax!

Holding muscles in a stretched position for a prolonged period of time causes the muscle spindles to become accustomed to the new length and stops them signalling. Training the stretch receptors is what stretching is all about.

There are many more receptors than spindle cells and golgi tendon receptors; they sense pressure, vibration, pain, position, direction and speed of motion. It is the combined input of all these receptors that influence the variety of reflex actions related to movement.

And it is this combination of normal reflexes that inhibit flexibility. So even though you can place one leg at right angles to your hips, when you try to do both together, as in side splits, the reflex contraction of the adductor muscles, stops you from doing so. A reflex we develop normally to prevent our legs from sliding apart when we walk.

The cure is simple. Un-do the normal reflex and you will be able to do side splits.

33

Inhibiting contraction

Different types of muscle contraction.

Isometric: this is a contraction where no movement takes place. An example of this would be pushing against a wall.

Isotonic: this is a contraction where movement does take place. An example of this would be lifting a weight.

Isotonic contractions can be further divided into concentric and eccentric contraction.

Concentric contraction is when the muscle becomes shorter.

Eccentric contraction is when the muscle becomes longer. An example of the two would be chin-ups; as the arms pull the body upwards the biceps are contracting concentrically, as the arms lower the body, the biceps are contracting eccentrically.

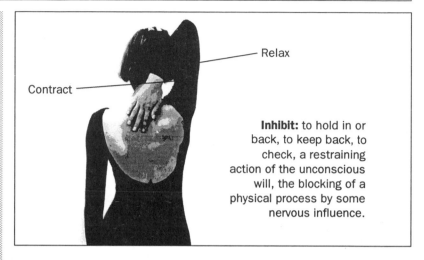

Contract

Relax

Inhibit: to hold in or back, to keep back, to check, a restraining action of the unconscious will, the blocking of a physical process by some nervous influence.

Muscles always work in groups. Since all that a muscle fibre can do is contract (it cannot actively lengthen), muscles usually work by opposing each other. One example is the bicep/tricep pair. When the bicep contracts, the arm bends and the tricep relaxes; when the tricep contracts, the arm straightens and the bicep relaxes.

In order for this to happen, the nervous system is arranged so that signals telling the bicep to contract inhibit the tricep and prevent it from contracting.

Definition of muscle groups.

Agonists/prime movers: these muscles cause movement to occur, they are primarily responsible for generating the normal range of movement in a joint.

Antagonists: these muscles work in opposition to the agonists and will return a limb to its original position.

Synergists: these muscles assist the agonists.

Fixators: these muscles provide support while a movement is taking place.

Brain-muscle links

The matrix of connective tissue that maintains the structure of your body was not created in isolation from your thoughts and emotions...

There is a small part of the brain called the cerebellum, which controls muscle tone, coordination and balance. Nerve fibres from the proprioceptors go to the cerebellum and some go to the cerebral cortex, (the part of the brain that is associated with conscious thought and emotions). So there is a continual flow of sensation to the brain and a continual flow of conscious and unconscious motor impulses coming from the brain.

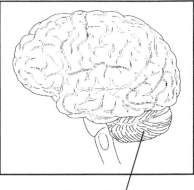
Cerebellum

Long term gains in flexibility depend on your ability to stretch the connective tissue binding your muscles, but your ability to do this is dependent upon your success in un-doing protective reflexes, and this in turn is related to your ability to relax mentally.

It is essential for you to realize that your state of mind and the force of your emotions can be even more difficult to overcome than the resistance of your muscles.

The matrix of connective tissue that maintains the structure of your body was not created in isolation from your thoughts and emotions, it was created simultaneously. Bear this in mind when you stretch. Be gentle, take it easy.

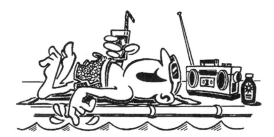

Stretching Without Pain

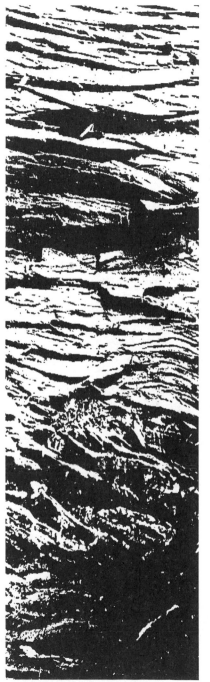

Mental and Emotional Aspects

Mental Connections

Concepts That Surround You

Head and neck
Shoulders
Arms/wrists and hands
Spine (cervical, thoracic and lumbar)
Hips
Legs
Ankles
Feet

Conclusion

Stretching Without Pain

Mental and Emotional Aspects

Flexibility is as much a state of mind as it is a condition of the body. The dictionary describes flexible as something that is easily bent. Another word that could be used is supple, which means pliant, lithe, yielding to the humour of others.

These words describe a complex interaction of connective tissue, physical sensation, emotions and thoughts which create the experience we call stretching. If you neglect the mental and emotional aspects, and concentrate only on the physical sensations it is like shutting the door in the face of your closest friends.

Most people know what it feels like to be tense. How certain muscles tighten until you feel like you are being gripped by a giant hand. How your breathing becomes shallow and unsatisfying. How your head pounds and your heart races....

And most people know what it feels like to be relaxed. How your muscles seem to fall into place. How your breathing deepens and refreshes you. How, even the blood flowing through your body creates a pleasant sensation of flowing warmth....

And what is it that creates these opposing conditions? Or aggravates one, or induces the other? It is your thinking.

This is generally understood to be true, but what is not so well understood is how specific and spatially located our thinking/feeling really is. That stiff neck—is it because you are unwilling to look at another's view point? Or the left hip that will not move properly—is it because you have trouble stepping away from what is familiar to you?

In this chapter we will explore some of these ideas. Stretch your mind a little.

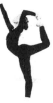

Mental Connections

The wise part is the part that knows something is possible, even though it may seem impossible right now.

Tension in the body always indicates some form of holding back, resistance, inability to let go. This is fairly obvious. What is not so obvious is that each area of the body has a specific relationship with certain mental and emotional states.

In other words, physical tension is directly related to mental/ emotional tension. And the physical location of this tension is directly related to its function in relation to you, as you *think* you are.

Stretching the body means increasing your normal range of motion. By trying to extend these 'normal' limits you begin to experience the way your muscles have been neurologically 'set.' The protective reflexes that you created in the first place, by trial and error, reinforce by action and sensation, these limits.

Transcending these limits sucessfully takes a united effort. Between the wise part of you, the talking part of you and the physical part of you. The wise part is the part that knows that something is possible, even though it may seem impossible right now. The talking part is the part that acts as an intermediary between the wise part and the physical body (which has its own rudimentary wisdom). And the physical part is like a partially domesticated animal, trained but wild at times.

The right approach is essential. In the past the animal part of you, which contains all of the hair-trigger protective reflexes, has been haphazardly programmed by a combination of acci- dents, some painful, some pleasurable. These accidentally created reflexes can be re-educated.

Remember, your natural flexibility is already considerable. The goal is simply to maximize what you already have. So start by considering your normal range of motion. When you find an area that seems restricted, also consider the way this lack of mobility affects your relationship with the external world.

**Concepts That
Surround You**

Head and neck

A flexible neck gives you the ability to look behind, in front, above and below. It supports your head and thus supports your thinking. Rigidity here indicates fixed vision. The muscles in this area control speaking and swallowing and the major blood vessels pass through this narrow supporting structure to nourish the brain. It is one of the more vulnerable parts of the body and usually contains a variety of over sensitive and mostly confused protective reflexes.

Shoulders

The shoulders are used for lifting, holding and carrying. Thus they are the areas associated with responsibility. Tight shoulders usually mean taking on too much, feeling overwhelmed and overloaded. Competitive athletes and dancers who are judged by their performance carry excessive amounts of self-imposed responsibility. Parental, peer and authority pressure adds to this. *The club / school / country / your future, depends on how well you perform.*

Arms/Wrists and Hands

The arms and hands are involved with holding and letting go, giving and receiving. The wrists allow you to do so with grace or clumsiness. At the wrist there is a condyloid joint, which closely mimics a ball and socket joint, affording almost a 360 degree range of motion. Stiffness here is associated with grasping and holding. Also the fear of letting go. Ask yourself, what are you afraid to hold on to, or let go of ?

Concepts That Surround You

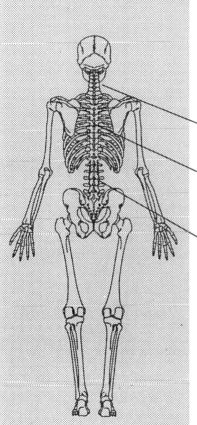

Spine

The spine supports and protects the spinal cord. The tension felt here is associated with harmony between the inside and outside. Between impulses coming from the central nervous system and moving towards the outside and impulses coming from outside and moving inwards. The spine also acts as an anchor point for many strong postural muscles which enable us to stand upright. It is a central, flexible axis that combines both form and movement.

Cervical spine: rigidity here relates to difficulty expressing yourself. Holding your voice inside. Stiff-necked, like a bull.

Thoracic spine: stiffness here is the fear of feeling emotion. Fear of life and of breathing and heart beat. Restricting what comes in and what goes out.

Lumbar spine: the personal power centre. Tension here means loss of connection with one's earth centre. This is the big shock absorber. If this area is stiff, then one's contact with the earth is harsh and unpleasant.

Hips

Control movement, forwards, backwards, side to side and up and down. Tension here means a reluctance to step out, to move away from one's centre. The sort of person who likes to get comfortable around well known objects or friends but does not like to move away from that place. Or feels very nervous when taken away from their safe space. Afraid of stepping in to the unknown. Uncomfortable with strong sexual sensations.

Concepts That Surround You

In general, the mental/ emotional problems associated with difficulty stretching certain areas of the body will either be past injuries that have re-set the muscle fibres with a feedback loop of pain sensations, thoughts and emotions that existed at the time, or faulty habits of working/thinking learned from observation or incorrect training. Continual stimulation of these areas will continue to strengthen the imbalance unless the training methods take into account all of the above factors.

Legs

Our legs carry us where we want to go. Being able to kick high means having the ability to use that strength to rise upwards. Jumping well depends on the flexibility of the calf muscles. Without this landings can be harsh and jarring. And take-offs will be stiff and unyielding. Our legs are the interface between us and the earth. Is our contact a pleasant or unpleasant experience? Stiff knees or weak knees indicate a lack of trust in one's ability to remain balanced while moving.

Ankles

Flexible but strong ankles enable you to adapt to a changing environment. The muscles here give you both speed and stamina. Similar to the wrists, the ankles provide suppleness and fine tuning of movement in relation to the earth and moving upon it. Imagine walking over rough ground with stiff ankles.

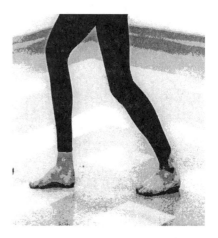

Feet

Give us our most continuous contact with the earth. Problems associated with stretching the feet often involve the desire to want to separate ourselves from the world. Like a soldier's boots are designed to protect him when he smashes his way through the world. Foot protection is only needed when there is force involved. Lack of trust that your feet will support you.

Concepts For Teachers

Treat muscles and connective tissue like you would treat a small child with a very limited vocabulary. Encouragement and warmth and creating a fascination for learning are the best techniques.

Over emphasis on competition will create a competitive attitude within as well as without. Rather than creating a will to win at all costs, why not encourage a passion to perform. There is a subtle difference. Passion is a burning desire associated with loving to do something because of the way you feel when you do it. Developing a competitive will means developing the attitude that there must always be a winner and a loser. This is essentially a divisive approach that leads to the eventual destruction of the person(s) involved.

An understanding of the mental/emotional connections can help teachers and coaches to understand a little more fully the processes involved in a person's life when they seem to be struggling with developing a certain area of their body.

Stretching, from the muscles' point of view, is letting go. Since muscles can only contract one of two ways, then this must be eccentric contraction (resisting lengthening).

Stretching, in terms of being able to reach farther, is a dynamic activity, balancing action with letting go. The prime mover or agonist, relies on the letting go of the antagonist.

The neurophysiology of stretching tells us that to become more flexible we need to re-educate our muscles, especially our protective reflexes. To enhance this process, I would add that we also need to learn why those reflexes were created in the first place.

Proprioception and the brain.

The cerebellum regulates muscle tone, coordination and balance. Other parts of the cerebral cortex are also associated with interpreting the sensations fed to it by the peripheral nervous system. These higher centres include areas of the brain which govern the emotions. And since these areas and the cerebellum are hard-wired, there can be little doubt that muscular tone and coordination are dependant on emotions and vice-versa.

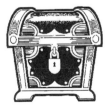

Conclusion

Flexibility is as much a state of mind as it is a condition of the body.

Transcending your limitations requires unity between your three parts: the wise part, the talking part and the physical part.

Concepts that surround you:
> Stiff-necked, bull-headed.
> Carrying the world on your shoulders.
> Limp-wristed or grasping.
> Spineless or stiff-backed.
> Tight-assed or shifty.
> Weak-kneed or legless.
> Feet of clay.

Passion—in the dictionary defined as an expression or outburst of feeling, an enthusiastic interest or direction of the mind.

Create within you a passion for extending yourself, for stretching your boundaries. Once this quality exists within you, the stretching of physical body parts becomes simple.

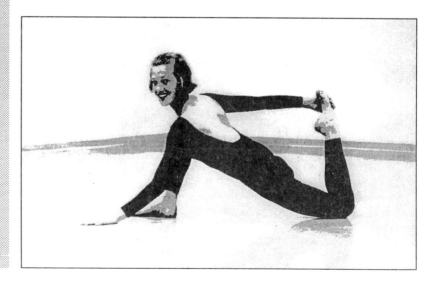

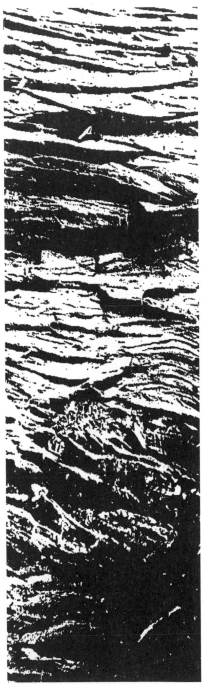

Warming Up

When to Stretch

Order of Stretching

Customize Your Stretching

Stretching Without Pain

Warming Up

Remember that stretching is not warming up!

Warming up means raising your body temperature one or two degrees. When you are warm you will automatically realize an increase in flexibility, without having done any stretching. This is because connective tissue becomes more flexible when it is warm.

The right kind of warm-up needs to be specific to the type of activity you wish to attempt. Dancers need to do a dance warm-up specific to the type of dance they are intending to practise. Gymnasts need to do a gym warm-up specific to the apparatus. Track athletes need to do their specific warm-up.

This is because the warm-up, as well as raising body temperature, is also preparing you by introducing you to the movements you are intending to perform a little later with full force.

At the end of your warm-up you should feel more alert, more coordinated and comfortably elastic. Your breathing should have deepened and your eyesight should have sharpened. You should not be tired after the warm-up.

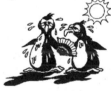

When to Stretch

The best time is when your muscles are warm.

However, you also need to take into account the weather or room temperature and the time of day. If the weather is cold, then you will usually need to warm-up longer before stretching. And generally it is easier to warm-up in the afternoon than in the morning.

But if you do train yourself to stretch in the morning (after a good warm-up) then you will find that it is even easier to stretch later on in the day. The morning stretches should be of a lesser intensity generally.

Order of Stretching

Something that is not well known, is that stretching in the correct order makes stretching easier.

Usually when you stretch you are stretching more than one muscle. You may try to isolate a particular muscle but there are always a collection of 'supporters' involved. These are usually the synergists.

So before stretching, for instance the hamstrings, you should stretch the synergists (gluteals, lower back, gastrocnemius, gracilis and sartorius). This way you have the whole group relaxed.

Information about muscle synergists related to specific muscles can be found in **The Muscle Book.** But actually it is quite easy to understand. Simply consider all the areas of tension felt when you attempt to do a specific stretch. If you want you can work from the extremities inwards towards the muscle you want to lengthen. Or work from either end of the muscle.

Generally you might want to work this way:

• stretch your upper and lower back
• stretch your sides
• stretch your arms before stretching your chest
• stretch your buttocks before stretching your groin
• stretch your calves before stretching your hamstrings
• stretch your shins before your quadriceps

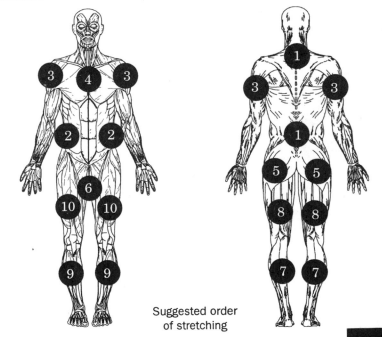

Suggested order of stretching

Stretch to Improve What You Do

Customize Your Stretching.

The connective tissue that surrounds and supports the muscle fibres grows in accordance with the tasks that the muscles are repeatedly asked to perform. In other words, if you do not stretch at all, the connective tissue will shrink to the length of the muscle fibre. If you have ever had a limb fixed in a cast you will know how tight unused muscles can become. Muscles that are not stretched will continue to try to contract.

It follows then that if you wish to perform an activity such as gymnastics or dance or martial arts, which demand a high level of dynamic flexibility (see Chapter 6), then you must train with dynamic flexibility exercises. Weight lifting followed by static stretching will not do the job.

The task of connective tissue is to act as a binding agent for muscle fibre (see Chapter 2, Fascia). It also enables the force of muscular contraction to act on either end (the origin and insertion) of the muscle.

If you wish to lift weights and do hundreds of repetitious movements within a short range of motion, you will not develop long, elastic muscles; you will develop short powerful muscles with a small range of movement. Static stretching after weight training does not alter the neuromuscular 'set' that you have created through this high intensity, short range activity.

Therefore your training program needs to include a variety of different types of stretches; dynamic, static, active and so on. The rule of thumb being if you want to be a dancer, then dance. If you want to be a weight lifter, then lift weights. If you want to have both strength and flexibility then you need to train strength through your entire range of motion.

And remember, ten minutes of stretching in the morning enables you to move through your full range of motion later in the day, *without an additional warm-up*. Because you have started the day telling your muscles–this is how long I want you to be all day!

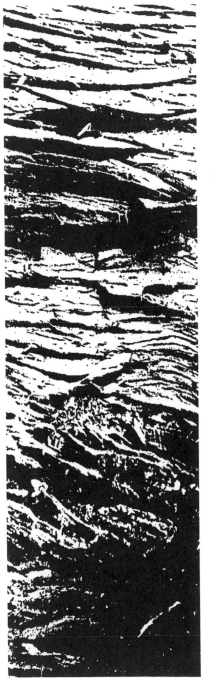

Stretching Techniques

Moving

Ballistic/elastic
Dynamic
Active

Non-moving

Passive
Static
Isometric
Proprioceptive Neuromuscular Facilitating

Types of Stretching

Moving:
ballistic/elastic
dynamic
active

Ballistics is bouncing—not really stretching at all.

Dynamic stretching is the sort you do naturally when you wake up in the morning.

There are two main categories of stretching, Moving and Non-moving.

Moving

Ballistic/Elastic

Ballistics is the study of projectiles. This type of limb-throwing is technically not stretching at all but describes how momentum is used to force a limb beyond its normal range of motion. It is sometimes called elastic stretching because of the bouncing motion involved. However, the speed of the movement only serves to activate the stretch reflexes which cause an involuntary tightening of the muscles, thereby cancelling any possibility of lengthening the tissues. It can also lead to injury and should never be attempted forcefully until the body is very warm.

Dynamic

This involves moving parts of the body and gradually increasing the range of motion and the speed or both. It is a controlled movement that takes you gently to the limits of your ability. There are no bouncy or jerking movements. An example of dynamic stretching would be slow, controlled leg, arm or torso movements.

Dynamic stretching is very useful as a part of the warm-up, especially if done as a series of repetitions. Repeat the movements until you feel slightly tired, then stop. Tired muscles are less elastic and if you continue to work them they will set a short-fibre memory into that movement, making it harder to lengthen the muscle the next time you try.

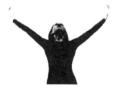

Active

This is also known as static-active stretching and is the type of movement where you assume a position and hold it. The action of the opposing muscles and the inhibitory factors involved help to train the muscles to relax and the antagonists to strengthen. An example of this would be lifting the leg to the front and holding it there. Active stretches are quite hard to hold for more than 10-15 seconds.

Non-moving

Passive/static

Also known as relaxed stretching or static-passive stretching. This describes the technique where you reach a position and hold it with another part of your body, or with a partner, or by using apparatus. Splits are an example of passive stretching, using the floor as the apparatus. If done slowly and in a relaxed manner this type of stretching is very good for cool down and to help reduce post-workout muscle fatigue.

Isometric

This is a type of static stretching which involves the resistance of muscle groups through tensing the stretched muscles.

This is one of the fastest ways to increase passive flexibility and it also helps to develop strength in the tensed muscles, which eventually helps active flexibility.

The resistance is applied away from the direction of movement. For example, if you are trying to stretch your hamstrings so that you can lift your leg higher to the front, you would tense the muscle (either against your arm, or with the help of another person, or a barre), by pushing downwards.

This type of stretching is not recommended for children and adolescents whose bones are still growing.

Active stretching depends on the strength of the prime mover.

Non-moving:
passive/static
isometric
PNF

Passive/static is the most common form of stretching.

Isometric contraction is when no movement takes place.

It is also recommended that isometric stretching be preceded by dynamic stretches. And that isometric stretching is not done more than once per day, per muscle group.

Procedure:
1. Assume the position of passive stretch.
2. Tense the stretched muscle for 7-15 seconds.
3. Relax the muscle for at least 20 seconds.

Isometric stretching works because it is a method of overcoming the stretch reflex by triggering the lengthening reflex. (See Chapter 3, Types of Muscle). This is how you 'train' your muscles to lengthen by re-educating the stretch reflex.

PNF

Is a method of combining passive and isometric stretching to achieve maximum static flexibility.

This technique was originally developed for injury rehabilitation.

What makes it different from isometric stretching is that after the contraction phase, the limb's range of movement is increased passively. This means that while the protective reflexes are 'turned off' the limb can be slowly moved into a new, extended position.

PNF = Proprioceptive Neuromuscular Facilitating.

Who ever thought up the name for this one must have been a serious techno-geek. Still, regardless of its name, it is the most effective stretching technique so far discovered.

PNF Procedure 1:

1. Assume the passive stretch position.
2. Isometrically tense the stretched muscle for 7-15 seconds.
3. Relax the muscle for 2-3 seconds.
4. Then immediately increase the passive stretch and hold for 10-15 seconds.
5. Relax for 20 seconds.

PNF Procedure 2:

1. Assume the passive stretch position.
2. Contract the stretched muscle isometrically for 7-15 seconds.
3. Contract the antagonist (the opposite muscle to the one being stretched) isometrically for 7-15 seconds.
4. Relax for 20 seconds.

Warning...

PNF stretching is not recommended for young children with growing bones. It is also not recommended to practise PNF stretching more than once per 36 hour period, per muscle group.

PNF stretching takes advantage of the fact that the reflex to contract a muscle at full stretch is turned off when the muscle contracts isometrically. The short time immediately after the contraction is the optimum time to train the stretch receptors into accepting a new increased range of muscle length.

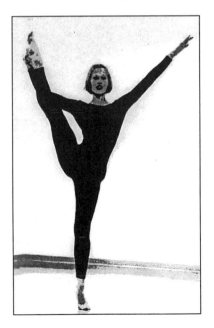

Stretching Without Pain

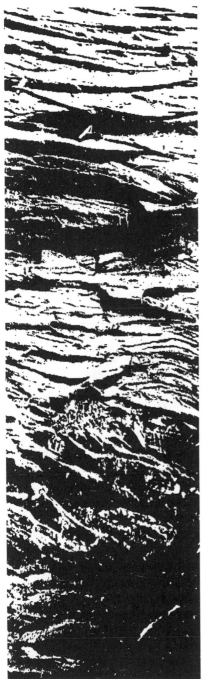

The Flexibility Supermarket

Neck
Shoulder
Arm, Elbow, Wrist
Spine
Hips
Leg, Knee, Ankle

Suggested Stretching Positions

Stretching Without Pain

The Flexibility Supermarket

The shoppers guide to stretching, including:

- the skeleton and joint structure
- the muscles
- mindbody
- danger spots.

The general areas covered will be:

- the neck
- shoulders
- arm, elbow, wrist
- spine
- pelvis
- leg, knee, ankle.

I am hoping that the following pages will enable you to visualize clearly the joints, muscles and connective tissue involved in each separate area of the body that you wish to stretch.

I have also included a few suggested stretching postures but I am more concerned that you understand firstly, the structure and function of the connective tissue you are stretching and secondly the principles involved in re-educating the muscles, by using gentle techniques to 'turn-off' the protective reflexes. Once these two concepts are firmly understood you will be able to create your own postures and methods to adapt to specific skills that you may be trying to develop.

In regard to the Mindbody information; these are guidelines or suggestions from my own experience both as a participant and as a therapist. The way you think about your body affects the way your body functions. Once you start to make connections between thinking and stretching, you will make much faster progress.

Enjoy!

Neck

Joint structure:
Cartilagenous joints.

Joint between skull and axis is a pivot joint..

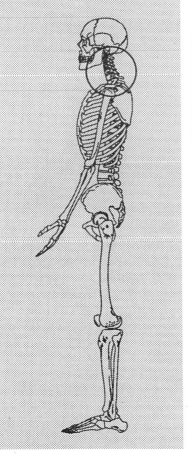

Muscles

Extensors (upper sacrospinalis group)

Flexors and rotators (sternocleidomastoid)

Side bending (upper trapezius, levator scapulae, sternocleidomastoid)

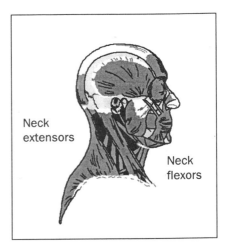

Neck extensors

Neck flexors

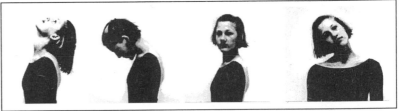

Mindbody

Freedom of movement here gives you the ability to look around; in front, behind, above, below and to either side. To see the world from a variety of viewpoints.

Lack of movement indicates a viewpoint restricted by excess tension and muscular armouring. Are you frightened to look around you?

Danger

This is one of the most vulnerable parts of the body. Forceful movements (such as whiplash) can easily damage the spinal cord, causing paralysis from the neck downwards. Stretching here should be done only to restore normal mobility.

Shoulder

Joint structure:
Synovial joint

Loose ball & socket.

Front view

Back view

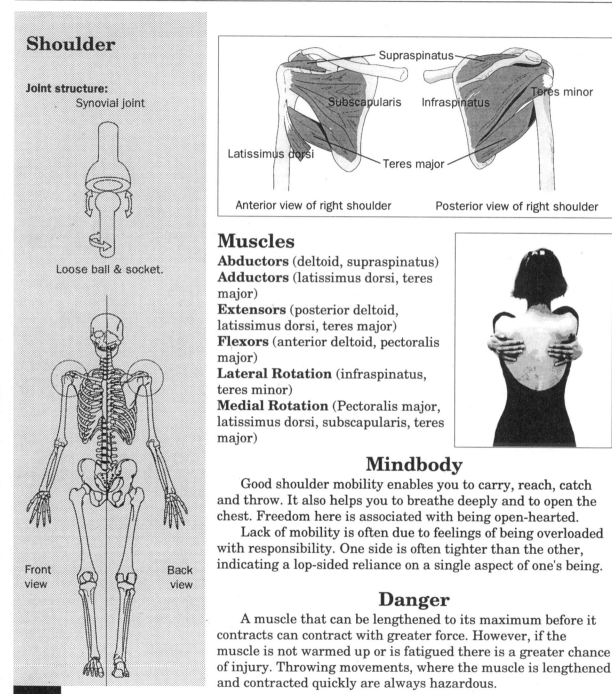

Supraspinatus

Subscapularis   Infraspinatus

Teres minor

Latissimus dorsi

Teres major

Anterior view of right shoulder   Posterior view of right shoulder

Muscles
Abductors (deltoid, supraspinatus)
Adductors (latissimus dorsi, teres major)
Extensors (posterior deltoid, latissimus dorsi, teres major)
Flexors (anterior deltoid, pectoralis major)
Lateral Rotation (infraspinatus, teres minor)
Medial Rotation (Pectoralis major, latissimus dorsi, subscapularis, teres major)

Mindbody
Good shoulder mobility enables you to carry, reach, catch and throw. It also helps you to breathe deeply and to open the chest. Freedom here is associated with being open-hearted.

Lack of mobility is often due to feelings of being overloaded with responsibility. One side is often tighter than the other, indicating a lop-sided reliance on a single aspect of one's being.

Danger
A muscle that can be lengthened to its maximum before it contracts can contract with greater force. However, if the muscle is not warmed up or is fatigued there is a greater chance of injury. Throwing movements, where the muscle is lengthened and contracted quickly are always hazardous.

Good shoulder mobility depends on three groups of muscle.

1. muscles that join the scapula to the arm
2. muscles that join the trunk to the scapula
3. muscles that join the trunk to the arm

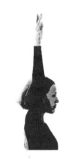

This is an example of static-active stretching for muscle groups 1, 2 & 3. Passive or isometric/PNF stretches can also be done in this position by leaning against a wall or chair with the torso at 90°.

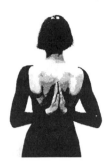

This position stretches groups 2 & 3 and is good for passive, isometric and PNF techniques.

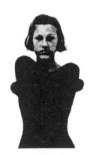

This stretch, which can be done passively or isometrically is excellent for stretching group 2 muscles.

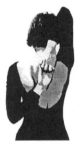

This position can be worked up to by using a towel or piece of wood to grasp. All the muscle groups are stretched. Alternate isometric/PNF stretching by first pulling with the upper arm and then pulling with the lower arm. This is a powerful stretch so go carefully at first.

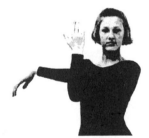

Stretching the arm across the front of the body and using the opposite arm for isometric or PNF stretching is a good way to stretch muscle groups 1 & 2.

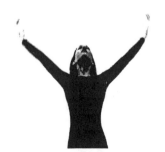

An example of dynamic stretching, swinging the arms slowly in gradually increasing circles. Good for all three muscle groups.

Stretching Without Pain

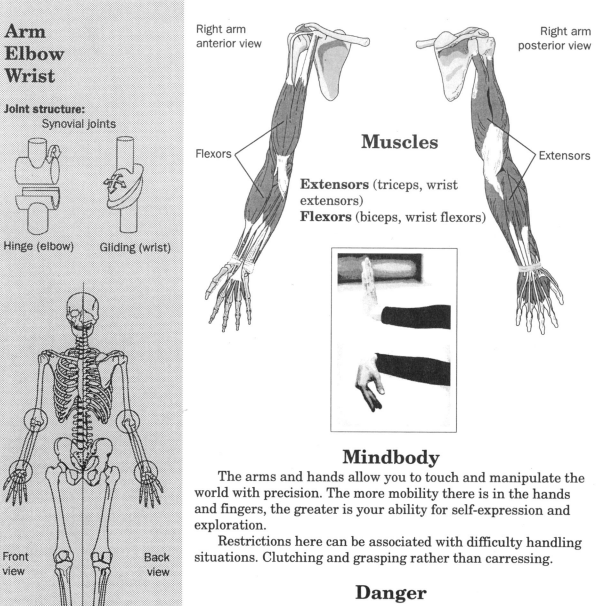

Arm Elbow Wrist

Joint structure:

Synovial joints

Hinge (elbow)   Gliding (wrist)

Front view   Back view

Right arm anterior view

Right arm posterior view

Flexors

Muscles

Extensors (triceps, wrist extensors)
Flexors (biceps, wrist flexors)

Extensors

Mindbody

The arms and hands allow you to touch and manipulate the world with precision. The more mobility there is in the hands and fingers, the greater is your ability for self-expression and exploration.

Restrictions here can be associated with difficulty handling situations. Clutching and grasping rather than carressing.

Danger

The wrists are the weak links, especially liable to injury from falling. Competitive cyclists are trained to roll onto their forearms and shoulders to avoid breaking these joints.

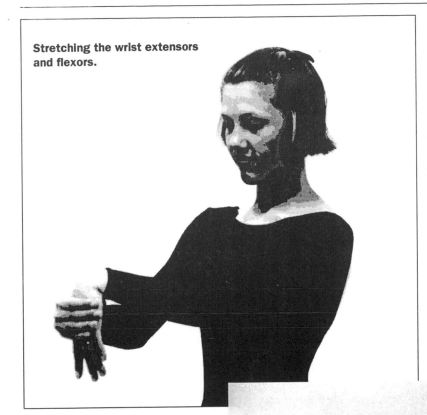

Stretching the wrist extensors and flexors.

This is the position to use when stretching the wrist flexors. Sports that utilize the forearm muscles such as badminton, squash, tennis and golf often lead to injuries such as tennis elbow or golfers elbow. The stress is on the origin of these muscles (which is the inner or outer portion of the humerus, depending on the muscle involved). Isometric and PNF stretching helps prevent excessive tension in these muscles.

To stretch isometrically simply hold the wrist in either the flexed or extended position, tense the muscles for 7-15 seconds, then relax. Repeat three times for each muscle group. The PNF method is to tense the muscle for 7-15 seconds, relax for 2-3 seconds then immediately increase the passive stretch and hold for a further 10-15 seconds. Then relax for 20 seconds. Repeat this no more than three times for each muscle group.

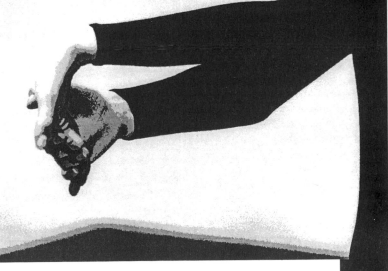

Spine

Joint structure:
Catilagenous joints

Partly moveable
(intervertebral)

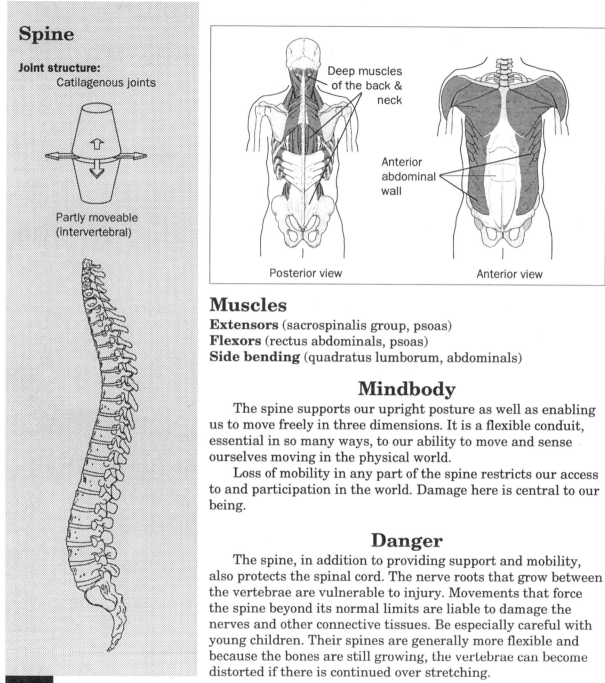

Deep muscles
of the back &
neck

Anterior
abdominal
wall

Posterior view

Anterior view

Muscles

Extensors (sacrospinalis group, psoas)
Flexors (rectus abdominals, psoas)
Side bending (quadratus lumborum, abdominals)

Mindbody

The spine supports our upright posture as well as enabling us to move freely in three dimensions. It is a flexible conduit, essential in so many ways, to our ability to move and sense ourselves moving in the physical world.

Loss of mobility in any part of the spine restricts our access to and participation in the world. Damage here is central to our being.

Danger

The spine, in addition to providing support and mobility, also protects the spinal cord. The nerve roots that grow between the vertebrae are vulnerable to injury. Movements that force the spine beyond its normal limits are liable to damage the nerves and other connective tissues. Be especially careful with young children. Their spines are generally more flexible and because the bones are still growing, the vertebrae can become distorted if there is continued over stretching.

The spine is a very complicated structure involving 7 cervical, 12 thoracic and 5 lumbar joints. Cartilagenous discs between the vertebrae act as shock absorbers and can become compressed by the loads we carry.

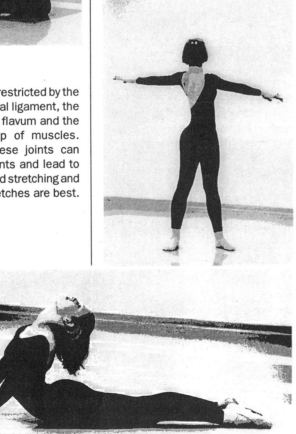

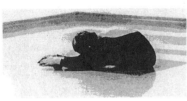

Forward bending is restricted by the posterior longitudinal ligament, the elastic ligamentum flavum and the sacrospinalis group of muscles. Over stretching these joints can weaken the ligaments and lead to disc injuries. Relaxed stretching and gentle dynamic stretches are best.

Rotation movements should be done slowly and in a relaxed manner. Above is a position that stretches many of the lower back and hip muscles. To the side is another method of stretching the whole spine but remember dynamic stretching means movement through the entire range of motion— NOT bouncing. Ballistic stretching in this position can be dangerous.

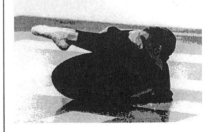

Curling the spine like this helps to relax the lumbar spine.

Extension movements as shown to the left, should be done with care, especially with young children, as the lumbar vertebrae and sacral joints can become over stretched and lead to an unstable spine.

Hips

Joint structure:
Synovial joint

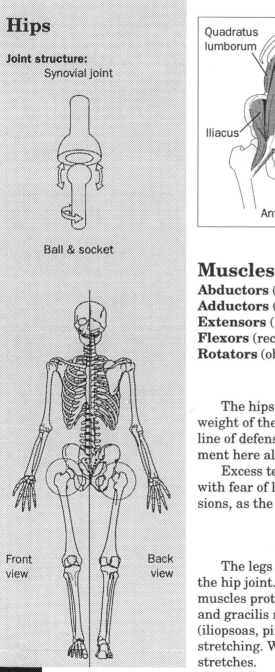

Ball & socket

Front view   Back view

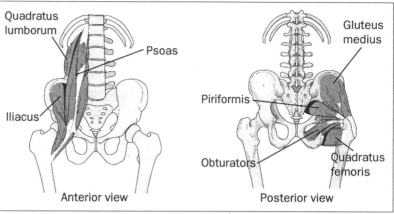

Quadratus lumborum
Psoas
Iliacus
Anterior view

Gluteus medius
Piriformis
Obturators
Quadratus femoris
Posterior view

Muscles

Abductors (gluteus medius/minimus, tensor fascia lata)
Adductors (adductors, gracilis)
Extensors (hamstrings, gluteus maximus)
Flexors (rectus femoris, iliopsoas, sartorius)
Rotators (obturators, piriformis, quadratus femoris)

Mindbody

The hips should be strong and flexible, spreading the weight of the torso evenly. Acting as a shock absorber, a first line of defense, protecting the lumbar spine. Freedom of movement here also permits healthy sexual sensations to arise.

Excess tension and rigidity in this area can be associated with fear of losing control. Also with difficulty making decisions, as the person shifts from side to side.

Danger

The legs are long levers which exert considerable force on the hip joint. This is why some of the strongest ligaments and muscles protect this area. Groin injuries involving the adductor and gracilis muscles are common. The deeper muscles, (iliopsoas, piriformis), are usually too tight and often need stretching. Work slowly developing both dynamic and static stretches.

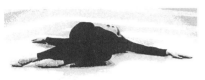

This position stretches the deep hip rotators as well as the gluteals and the long fascial sheath that runs down the outside of the thigh.

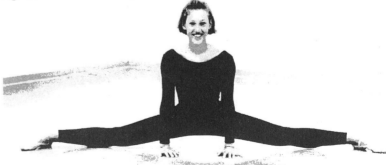

Preparation for the front splits begins with the top position. With the knees bent you can see that the 180° position of the legs is not difficult. Isometric and PNF stretching begins here, gradually straightening the knees as you progress.

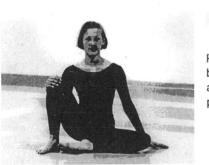

Note the angle of the left hip and thigh. By not engaging the right adductors, there is no protective resistance to fight against. However, in the picture below the arms are needed to press down on the thighs because the normal muscle reflexes are to pull the legs towards each other. This is an excellent posture for isometric and PNF stretches. Resistance is against the arms.

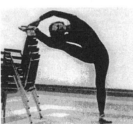

Side splits are only possible when the legs are rotated outwards or the pelvis is tilted forwards. For a gymnast to do a side split on a balance beam the pelvis needs to be tilted forwards so that the feet can stay on the beam. But for a dancer to achieve a position with the leg lifted to the side, the leg needs to be outwardly rotated.

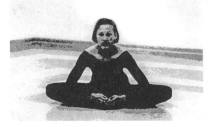

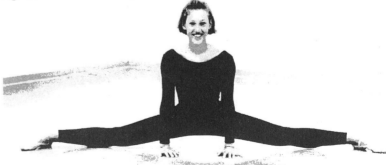

Leg
Knee
Ankle

Joint structure:

Synovial joints

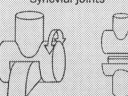

(ankle)   Hinge   (knee)

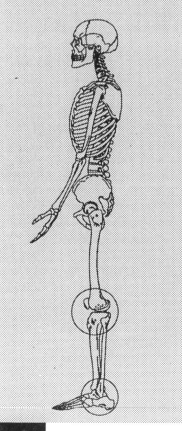

Muscles

Extensors (quadriceps, anterior tibials and ankle extensors)
Flexors (hamstrings, soleus, gastrocnemius)

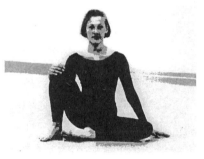

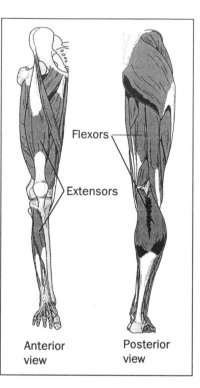

Flexors

Extensors

Anterior view

Posterior view

Mindbody

The knees and ankles allow us to accept change rapidly, without losing balance. They allow us to adapt to a variety of different surfaces, to stand tall when necessary; or to stoop low, when appropriate.

Stiff knees and ankles indicate a certain amount of stubbornness, an unwillingness to bend. An inflexible stance taken.

Danger

The knees and ankles are susceptible to torsion. Both joints are hinges and they do not like to be twisted. These joints should be both strong and supple. Easily bent but not weak. Be especially careful when the muscles are cold or tired.

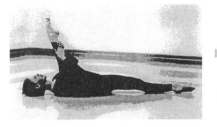

Hamstring stretch with the knee bent—note there is ample hip mobility.

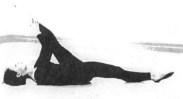

Hamstring stretch with the knee straight and the foot pointed.

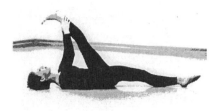

Hamstring stretch with the knee straight and the ankle dorsi-flexed. Note how the calf muscle affects hip flexibility.

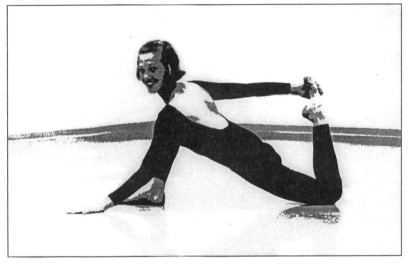

This is an excellent way of stretching the quadriceps and psoas muscles. To stretch isometrically, push against the hand with the foot. Some padding under the knee is helpful.

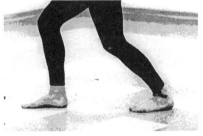

Position for stretching the soleus (deep calf) muscle.

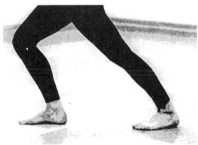

Position for stretching the gastrocnemius (surface calf) muscle. The two positions to the left are also for stretching the calf muscles. The far left for the deep calf and the near left for the surface calf. Stretch these before the hamstrings.

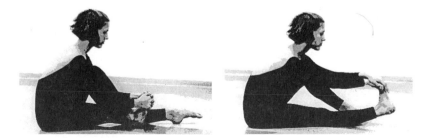

67

Stretching Without Pain

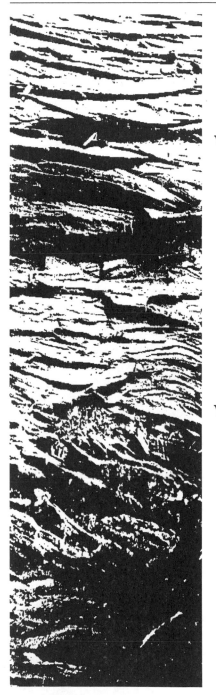

War Zones

Eyes, forehead, temple, back of head
Jaw, ears, base of skull
Neck
Upper chest, shoulders, upper back
Chest, ribs, shoulder blades
Diaphragm, lower ribs
Abdomen, lower back
Lower abdomen, hips, buttocks
Peripheral zones:
    elbow
    wrist
    knee
    ankle

What Has This to do With Stretching?

Stretching Without Pain

War Zones

In Chapter 4 we looked at the Concepts That Surround You. In this chapter we will be examining what I call War Zones—areas of the body that create rings of tension. These areas are important because they tend to be reservoirs of chronic rigidity. And since the ability to stretch freely depends largely on the ability to relax, these stress reservoirs act like knots, restricting the free flow of energy within the body.

Starting at the Top

First zone: eyes, forehead, temples and back of the head. This relates to seeing, or not seeing. And thinking, particularly the ability to concentrate. The war between what is seen, what you would like to see, and what you think you are seeing. Fear of seeing something awful.

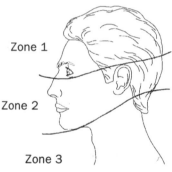

Second zone: the jaw, ears and base of the skull. Controlling one's speech, or not being able to control speech creates tension in this area. Hearing and speaking, knowing when to listen and when to talk. The war of control. Fear of the loss of control.

Third zone: the neck. Tension here acts like a noose, preventing air from entering and exiting the body. It is where we allow in what we need and allow out what we no longer need. The war for access to the body. The fear of possession. The breath-funnel and the swallowing tube. Being able to express yourself, or not being able to let out your feelings. Can you sing, can you shout—or do you squeak when you speak ?

War Zones

In the Middle

Fourth zone: upper chest, shoulders and upper back. Relates to the shouldering of burdens and responsibilities. This is where your conscience sits, hopping from one shoulder to the other, using the voice of your father or mother to admonish you. Fear of not doing one's duty. Of failing.

Fifth zone: chest, ribs and shoulder blades. The heart centre. Where we feel love. Or where we armour ourselves so that we do not have to feel love, or the pain of not being loved, or falling out of love.

The sixth zone: diaphragm and lower ribs. Control of the breath. If this zone is tense there is a fear of letting go, particularly in relation to strong emotions. Having to do with personal needs and desires. The war for nourishment and personal pleasure. The fear of not having enough. Of not being able to breathe deeply, to take in enough of what you want and to get rid of what you no longer need.

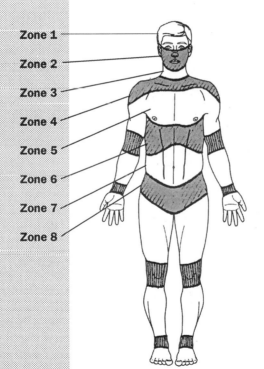

Zone 1
Zone 2
Zone 3
Zone 4
Zone 5
Zone 6
Zone 7
Zone 8

War Zones

Lower Parts and Extremities

Seventh zone: abdomen and lower back. Tension here relates to an attempt to control personal power. It is the location of your earth centre and when this area is relaxed you will feel connected to your environment. A sense of belonging and acceptance. Stiffness here indicates a lack of self-trust or lack of knowledge of purpose.

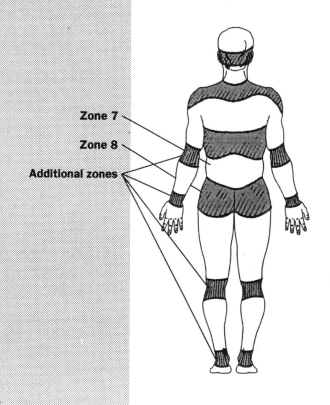

Zone 7

Zone 8

Additional zones

Eighth zone: lower abdomen, hips and buttocks. The area of sexual energy and of letting go through the process of urination and defecation. The war here is for release, discharge. The fear is of letting go.

Additional zones: can be found encircling the arms, (elbows and wrists) and legs, (knees and ankles). Individual fingers and joints also create zones as do the articulations of the feet. These extremity zones are usually related to either zone 4 (arms) or zone 8 (legs). Thus arms are associated with dealing with burdens and responsibilities and the legs with powerful sexual and creative energies.

War Zones

Elbow, Wrist, Knee, Ankle

The elbow war zone is associated with the ability to bring toward or to push away.

The wrist zones are associated with being able to manipulate objects in circles. Tension in the elbows or wrists will be associated with some aspect of shoulder or neck war (relating to the responsibility).

The knee war zone is associated with being able to stand firmly, but with resilience.

The ankle zones are associated with being able to sense the ground. Difficulties in either of these areas relates to hip dysfunctions associated with letting go. The inability to feel grounded is not being able to let gravity go through the body.

Extremity war zones are almost always associated with trunk segment war zones. The trunk zones are designed to rotate around body centres. But if these trunk segments become rigid, the rotation around the centre is diminished and a state of stagnation develops. This leads to a reduction of energy to the extremities and subsequent loss of sensation and control.

What has this to do with stretching?

Now you might ask, "What has this to do with stretching ?"

If you look back to the first pages of this book you will see that you have travelled from joint structures, ranges of motion, connective tissues, the mechanisms that cause muscles to contract, mental-emotional aspects, warm-up advice, stretching techniques and finally to the flexibility supermarket. Gradually moving from microscopic muscle fibres to an overview of the body as a whole. And finally to war zones. A concept of interrelatedness in an easy to remember package.

Stretching Without Pain

Recognizing a war zone for what it is, is the first step towards being able to release the neuromuscular programming that maintains it.

Just as there are areas of the world that have been 'hot-spots' for centuries due to a geography and climate that leads to conflict, so there are areas of the body that are liable to greater concentrations of stress.

Remember that each of the war zone segments is comprised of groups of muscles acting as agonist/antagonist and that when you stimulate one muscle you also activate the various protective reflexes and inhibitory mechanisms of all the other related muscles.

By recognizing these war zones and by intelligent stretching of areas of rigidity, whole segments of the body can be released.

And careful analysis can lead to an understanding of why one person has difficulty stretching the neck and shoulder muscles, while being perfectly flexible in the hips and lower back. Over burdened with responsibility perhaps but able to discharge much of the pressure through the legs. Make a good runner, but might have difficulty doing gymnastics—won't be able to withstand the pressure.

It is a useful exercise to compare the tight areas of your body in relation to your life to date. Which war zones are activated ? And when you start to stretch this area, do you start to see those aspects of your life in a different light ?

An example from my own life:

I was attempting to choreograph a 20 minute dance work, with nine dancers. The music I had chosen contained a variety of complicated rhythms and some of the dancers had difficulty learning the steps, which meant that much of our rehearsal time was spent repeating moves that I thought they should be able to pick up quickly. In addition, our rehearsal time was at the end of a long day, so most of them were exhausted by the time I got them. And to top it off, one dancer decided to utilize the time to act out a bewildering number of personal problems. Needless to say, I became more and more frustrated.

Zone two is the jaw, ears and base of the skull.

Zone three is the neck.

Zone four is the upper chest, shoulders and upper back.

But instead of expressing my displeasure and concern, I allowed it to ferment inside. Which resulted in my upper back, right shoulder and neck locking in a severe spasm.

Visits to the chiropractor helped but it wasn't until I started yelling that the worst of the spasm began to release.

The war zones worst affected were two, three and four. Controlling speech, not expressing myself and shouldering too much responsibility.

Restoring normal mobility took several months—fortunately I knew how to stretch.

I hope the information in this book will enable you to avoid some of the school-of-hard-knocks that I have had to endure and that it will allow you to understand firstly *what you are stretching*, secondly *how to stretch it,* and thirdly *why you are stretching*.

**Relax,
take
it
easy.**

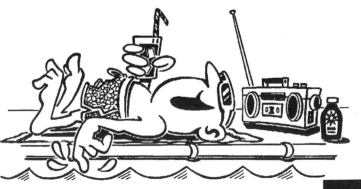

Bibliography

Athletic Ability & the Anatomy of Motion: Rolf Wirhed; Wolfe Medical Publications 1984; ISBN 0 7234 0854 8

Gray's Anatomy: Henry Gray, FRS; Crown Publishers Inc 1977; ISBN 0 517 223651

Physical Examination of the Spine and Extremities: Stanley Hoppenfeld MD; Appleton-Century-Crofts 1976; ISBN 0 8385 7853 5

Sports Injuries, Their prevention and treatment: Dr Lars Peterson and Dr Per Renström; Martin Dunitz Ltd 1986; ISBN 0 906348 91 9

Stretching and Flexibility, Everything you never wanted to know: Brad Appleton; Internet 1993; via anonymous ftp from host [cs.huji.ac.il] under the directory /pub/doc/faq/rec/martial.arts

Stretching Scientifically, a guide to flexibility training: Thomas Kurz MSc; Stadion Publishing Company 1991; ISBN 0 940149 28 1

Structural Fitness: John L Stirk; Elm Tree Books 1988; ISBN 0 241 12431 X

Textbook of Anatomy & Physiology: Anthony and Thibodeau; The C V Mosby Company 1983; ISBN 0 8016 0289 0

Textbook of Massage: L L Despard; Oxford University Press 1914

The Anatomy Colouring Book: Wynn Kapit/Lawrence M Elson; Harper & Row 1977; ISBN 0 06 453914 8

The Joy of Feeling: Iona Marsaa Teeguarden; Japan Publications Inc 1991; ISBN 0 87040 634 5

The Muscle Book: Paul Blakey; Bibliotek Books 1992; ISBN 1 873017 00 6